REVERSING

PREDIABETES:

The Comprehensive Guide to Reversing Insulin Resistance Naturally

JOHN M. WESTERN

TABLE OF CONTENT

INTRODUCTION

Do you count among the 88 million adult Americans who have prediabetes? If this is the case, you could be blissfully oblivious to the fact that your body is clearly alerting you. The good news is that prediabetes is a significant metabolic disease that requires careful attention. Prediabetes, in contrast to type 2 diabetes, is often curable with good lifestyle choices. This implies that you have a fantastic chance to take charge of your health before more serious problems arise.

Describe prediabetes.

Higher than usual blood sugar levels are indicative of prediabetes, but they are not yet high enough to be classified as type 2 diabetes. It indicates that, for a fasting blood glucose test, your blood sugar levels are between 100 and 125 mg/dL, and for an oral glucose tolerance test, they are between 140 and 199 mg/dL. Your body finds it difficult to properly control insulin so that it can metabolize the glucose that you ingest.

For most people, prediabetes is a warning indicator that, if treatment is ignored, type 2 diabetes will probably develop soon. Within ten years, a startling 70% of individuals with prediabetes will get type 2 diabetes. What's more scary is that 90% of people are thought to be unaware that they have this silent illness developing already.

The Dangers and Issues of Ignoring Pre-Diabetes
It would be quite expensive to ignore prediabetes as "no big deal" for your life and

health. Even before type 2 diabetes manifests, prediabetes may harm every part of the body. It may lead to erectile dysfunction, renal illness, nerve damage, eyesight loss, and other severe consequences. It also quickens the onset of heart disease and raises the risk of stroke.

Even if you are just in the prediabetes stage, your chances of developing:

- Cardiovascular disease: Compared to those with normal blood sugar levels, individuals with prediabetes have a roughly 50% increased risk of having cardiovascular disease.

- Neuropathy: Since 1 in 4 prediabetic individuals already have neuropathy that has been proven, there is a very real risk that prediabetes may damage nerves.

- Non-alcoholic fatty liver disease: This condition, which may result in cirrhosis and liver failure, is present in up to 70% of individuals with prediabetes.

- Cancer: Having prediabetes raises the risk of breast, colorectal, and pancreatic cancers, among other malignancies.

If left untreated, prediabetes eventually robs you of your vigor, independence, and overall health. It's a warning indication of much greater death rates from heart disease and cancer.

The Amazing Advantages of Treating Prediabetes

Reversing prediabetes has amazing benefits, despite the frightening hazards of continuing to be prediabetic. After changing their lifestyles, more than one in four individuals with prediabetes had normal blood sugar levels in only a year. These identical changes may, for many, permanently improve your body's capacity to use insulin as intended and sustain stable blood sugar levels.

Reversing your prediabetes can allow you to significantly lower or completely prevent your chances of:

Type 2 diabetes and its potentially fatal side effects
Heart disease and stroke; neuropathy and nerve damage; kidney disease; fatty liver disease; Alzheimer's disease and cognitive

decline; pancreatic, colon, and breast cancers; vision loss and blindness

In addition to avoiding these fatal chronic illnesses, you'll experience stable blood sugar levels, shed extra pounds, become less dependent on medicine, and develop a whole new perspective on living a vibrant life. You may live longer and look younger if you take control of your prediabetes.

This book will walk you through the entire process of resetting your body, using evidence-based dietary and lifestyle modifications that have helped thousands of people restore their health. You'll discover how to use food as a tasty medication, how to treat insulin resistance with basic workout techniques, and how to effectively de-stress for improved metabolic performance. It's time to take control of your prediabetes and ensure a robust, healthy life you can enjoy for decades to ahead. Stop worrying about the future and what may go wrong.

Chapter 1:

Prediabetes Explained

It's important to first comprehend precisely what prediabetes is, how it's diagnosed, and how it differs from type 2 diabetes before we can discuss how to cure it. Gaining a firm understanding of these principles will enable you to behave with purpose.

Criteria for Diagnosis and Definition

When blood sugar levels are higher than usual but not high enough to be classified as type 2 diabetes, it is called prediabetes, a dangerous metabolic illness. It is essentially an insulin-resistant condition of reduced glucose tolerance.

The body can effectively employ the hormone insulin in a person without prediabetes to control blood sugar levels within a healthy range. Cells may either store glucose for later use or utilize it as energy thanks to insulin.

Insulin resistance begins to develop with prediabetes. Insulin-induced cell resistance inhibits the body's ability to properly metabolize glucose. As a result, glucose accumulates in the circulation over time rather than being taken up by cells.

The pancreas works extra hard to compensate by increasing the amount of insulin it produces. When it eventually isn't able to meet the demand, the blood still contains extra glucose.

It is this persistently high blood sugar that is known as prediabetes.

To identify prediabetes, there are three primary tests performed:

1. Fasting plasma glucose test: You have prediabetes if your fasting blood sugar is between 100 and 125 mg/dL. The typical range for fasting is <100 mg/dL.

2. Oral glucose tolerance test: A blood sugar level of 140–199 mg/dL two hours after consuming a sugary beverage is indicative of prediabetes. Less than 140 mg/dL is normal.

3. A1C test: This gives you an average blood sugar reading over a period of two to three months. An A1C between 5.7%

and 6.4% indicates prediabetes. 5.7% and below is typical.

It is concerning if any of those test findings falls into the prediabetic category. Nonetheless, a mixture of borderline prediabetes values is often seen. For example, a person may have an A1C of 6.1% with a fasting glucose of 100 mg/dL.

If you have a family history of diabetes, are overweight, have high blood pressure, high triglycerides, or any of these conditions, it's important to be checked yearly. Your greatest chance of treating prediabetes and avoiding type 2 diabetes in the future is to take action as soon as possible.

Type 2 Diabetes vs Prediabetes

The degree of insulin resistance and degree of blood sugar rise are the primary distinctions between prediabetes and type 2 diabetes. The pancreas still produces enough insulin to maintain blood sugar levels below the diabetic threshold even while insulin resistance is growing in prediabetes. Insulin resistance has become much worse in type 2 diabetes, and the pancreas can no longer produce enough insulin to get over it.

The following blood sugar levels are necessary to diagnose type 2 diabetes:

- Blood sugar level after fasting 126 mg/dL or more
- A glucose tolerance test result of 200 mg/dL or above after two hours
- 6.5% or above for the A1C

These figures are considerably higher than prediabetes ranges, as you can see. When substantial insulin resistance has led to additional dysregulation of blood sugar, type 2 diabetes is diagnosed.

Unchecked prediabetes will ultimately lead to increased insulin resistance, which will cause type 2 diabetes in many individuals within ten years. In reality, studies reveal that in the absence of treatment, 70% of prediabetics would become type 2 diabetes.

Reversing type 2 diabetes is much more difficult than reversing prediabetes, even if it is doable in some situations. Making good lifestyle choices, like as eating a balanced diet and exercising often, may help restore insulin sensitivity and return blood sugar levels to normal when a person is in the prediabetes stage.

Reasons and Danger Elements

It is useful to examine the underlying causes and contributors of insulin resistance in order to better understand how prediabetes develops and your individual risk factors. Although genetics can play a part, prediabetes is often a disease that can be prevented and treated by a combination of lifestyle factors.

The following are the two main causes of insulin resistance:

1. Being overweight or obese: Carrying extra weight around the abdomen, in particular, is a major cause of insulin resistance. The hormones and other

substances produced by fat cells have the direct potential to obstruct insulin's capacity to appropriately control blood sugar levels.

2. Sedentary lifestyle/inactivity: Over time, your body's muscle cells develop resistant to insulin if you don't engage in regular physical activity. Muscles' capacity to absorb glucose in response to insulin is reduced when they are not in use.

In addition to weight and inactivity, a number of other variables may worsen insulin resistance and raise the risk of prediabetes, such as:

- **Diet:** An excessive intake of processed foods and refined carbohydrates may cause blood sugar and insulin levels to increase often, which can contribute to insulin resistance. Low fiber consumption might potentially be a factor.

- **Sleep problems:** It has been shown that insufficient sleep impairs insulin sensitivity and blood sugar metabolism.

- **Chronic stress:** Insulin's ability to function normally may be hampered by stress hormones like glucagon and cortisol.

- **Smoking:** It has been shown that the chemicals in cigarette smoke directly affect how well insulin functions inside cells.

- **Genetics:** You are more likely to develop insulin resistance if you have a family history of diabetes. A increased risk also affects certain ethnic groups, such as Asian Americans, Hispanics, and African Americans.

- **Age:** As we age, insulin resistance tends to naturally rise; by their 60s and 70s, most individuals have some level of age-related insulin resistance.

Additional medical conditions: High blood pressure, sleep apnea, non-alcoholic fatty liver disease, and polycystic ovarian syndrome (PCOS) might all be factors.

The good news is that a lot of these risk factors for prediabetes may be altered by making dietary and lifestyle adjustments. One of the most effective strategies to improve insulin sensitivity and stop or treat prediabetes is to maintain a healthy weight via food and exercise.

The first step towards implementing remedial action is realizing that prediabetes is a significant but often treatable illness. You are now able to take control of your health by making educated decisions since you understand what it is, how it's diagnosed, and what variables raise your risk. The precise food, exercise, and lifestyle choices that have been shown to reverse prediabetes will be covered in detail in the next chapters.

Chapter 2:

Blood Sugar Regulation

Understanding the body's complex blood sugar management system is essential to understanding prediabetes and how to reverse it. Knowing this will enable you to understand the starting point of insulin resistance's metabolic malfunction and the significance of maintaining normal blood sugar levels for general health.

The Functions of Blood Sugar

The main energy source for every cell in your body is glucose. It's a simple sugar that's produced when your food's carbs are broken down. Your circulation carries glucose, which cells in your muscles, tissues, and other organs need as fuel.

But glucose can't just go right through cell membranes by itself. Insulin is a strong hormone that is necessary for cells to effectively absorb and digest glucose.

The pancreas, which constantly checks blood sugar levels, produces insulin via beta cells. Following a carbohydrate-rich meal, the pancreas gets signals to begin releasing bursts of insulin into the circulation as blood glucose begins to rise.

The key that opens cells to let glucose in is insulin. By binding to receptors on the surfaces of cells, it functions as a shuttle, directing those cells to take up and process glucose from the bloodstream for storage or energy. In the absence of insulin, glucose becomes trapped outside of cells, where it circulates uncontrollably and accumulates to potentially hazardously high blood levels.

Within two hours of eating, insulin has assisted in moving enough glucose into cells so that, once digestion is finished, blood sugar levels begin to fall back to their pre-meal levels. At your subsequent carb-containing meal or snack, the cycle is repeated.

You may safely enjoy meals rich in carbohydrates thanks to this sophisticated insulin-glucose management system, which also guards against dangerous blood sugar fluctuations or persistently high blood sugar levels that over time may harm cells and organs. Blood sugar levels stay within a safe range as long as insulin is functioning as it should.

Resistance to Insulin

The underlying cause of type 2 diabetes and prediabetes is insulin resistance. In this condition, cells lose their ability to react effectively to insulin's instructions, which stops glucose from being digested correctly.

The precise processes that lead to insulin resistance are complicated and not entirely known. However, studies reveal that this malfunction is often brought on by two major drivers:

1. Being overweight or obese - Hormones and other chemicals produced by adipose tissue, or fat cells, have the

direct ability to disrupt insulin signaling pathways. The degree of insulin resistance increases with the amount of extra fat stored, particularly around abdominal organs.

2. Inactivity - Over time, muscles that do not contract as a result of physical activity develop insulin resistance. Since contraction of muscles facilitates the absorption of glucose, sedentary muscles become less responsive to insulin.

Apart from these variables, over time, persistent unhealthy behaviors such as smoking, stress, sleep deprivation, and poor food may worsen insulin resistance by causing mitochondrial dysfunction and inflammatory pathways.

Blood sugar levels may stay mostly normal when insulin resistance first appears because the pancreas produces extra insulin to make up for it. Imagine applying more pressure to the gas pedal to overcome the resistance, but the vehicle (the cells) continues to move.

But the pancreas is limited in its ability to produce extra insulin at this level forever. Eventually, beta cells wear out and become depleted. When insulin levels fall, blood sugar levels rise and glucose cannot enter cells as effectively; this is the start of prediabetes.

Making dietary and lifestyle modifications to lessen insulin resistance is now essential. Insulin resistance gradually develops into type 2 diabetes if it doesn't get better. Because there is too much insulin resistance for the pancreas to overcome with its diminishing insulin production, dangerously high blood sugar levels continue to exist.

Additional Hormones At Play

Insulin is the primary modulator of glucose metabolism, however it is not the only factor. Other hormones that contribute to blood sugar control and energy balance include the following:

- **Glucagon:** This hormone tells the liver to release glucose that has been stored in the body in between meals, working against insulin's effects. Glucagon levels in diabetics are often comparatively low.

- **Amylin:** Amylin, which is secreted in tandem with insulin, helps control the rate at which food passes through the digestive system and conveys the sensation of fullness or satisfaction. In those with diabetes, it is compromised.

- **GLP-1:** After meals, the stomach secretes an incretin hormone that increases insulin release and suppresses glucagon secretion. High blood sugar may be a result of impaired GLP-1.

Epinephrine, often known as adrenaline, is a fight-or-flight hormone that causes a spike in blood sugar and blocks the release of insulin to give you a surge of energy when you're under severe stress. Long-term stress raises blood sugar levels.

The main stress hormone, cortisol, interferes with insulin action and production, gradually leading to an increase in insulin resistance.

Growth hormone: By opposing insulin, this pituitary hormone aids in the process known as gluconeogenesis, which gives cells more energy. Elevations may indicate increased blood sugar levels.

Insulin keeps blood sugar within a reasonable level when all these hormones are in perfect balance. However, poorly controlled diabetes and prolonged insulin resistance lead to hormonal dysregulation and malfunction.

When a person is diagnosed with prediabetes, there is still time to make lifestyle changes that will increase insulin sensitivity and prevent a hormonal storm that would cause metabolic instability and persistently high blood sugar levels.

Comprehending the physiological processes behind insulin resistance and blood sugar homeostasis provide the fundamental understanding needed to begin the reversal of prediabetes. You will learn in detail in the next chapters how to use food, exercise, and other variables to reset this hormonal balance and take back control of your blood sugar management.

Chapter 3:

Dietary Strategies

The amount of blood sugar and insulin that your body can control is greatly influenced by the food you consume. Insulin resistance may be exacerbated by certain foods and dietary habits, which can raise blood sugar and prolong the cycle of prediabetes. On the other hand, one of the most effective methods to improve insulin sensitivity and treat prediabetes is by deliberate dietary modifications.

This chapter will go over precise, research-backed dietary methods for controlling blood sugar, boosting foods that help optimize your consumption of carbohydrates, and managing your weight using portion control. Reversing prediabetes requires sustained dietary modifications.

Low-Glycemic vs. Low-Carb Diets

Cutting down on all carbs, especially refined and processed carbs, is one of the best dietary strategies for treating type 2 diabetes and prediabetes. This lessens the total amount of glucose that your body must process.

Very low-carb diets limit the amount of carbohydrates to 20% of calories or less, whereas low-carb diets are defined as obtaining fewer than 30% of total calories from carbohydrates. Low-starch veggies, low-sugar fruits, healthy fats, and proteins are among the items that should be prioritized.

Compared to low-fat, higher-carb diets, low-carb diets are more successful in improving insulin sensitivity, lowering blood sugar and A1C levels, and improving insulin sensitivity in those with type 2 diabetes and prediabetes. The advantages often increase with the degree of carbohydrate restriction.

Some people, however, find very low-carb diets to be too restrictive and challenging to stick to over time. An alternative is to stick to a low-glycemic diet that minimizes the pace at which carbs are absorbed.

Foods containing carbohydrates are ranked from 0 to 100 on the glycemic index (GI) according to how they affect blood sugar levels. High GI foods include potatoes, refined grains, sugary snacks, and sweets. These foods can induce sharp rises in blood sugar levels. Low-GI meals, on the other hand, have a slow, regulated influence on blood sugar.

Foods low in GI include:

- Vegetables that aren't starchy
- Pulses and legumes
- Berries
- Almonds and their butters

- Whole grains, such as steel- Sprouting grain bread and chopped oats - Dairy items such as cottage cheese and yogurt

Maintaining blood sugar management while creating a diet that is more sustainable for some individuals may be achieved by distributing your carbohydrate consumption among a variety of low-glycemic meals as well as healthy proteins and fats. It has been shown that focusing on meals with a low GI load reduces insulin resistance.

Cutting down on the quantity of quickly absorbed carbohydrates in your diet may help avoid blood sugar spikes and the crashes that follow, whether you choose to follow a very low-carb diet or only stick to low-GI carb sources. Your pancreas's need to continuously secrete insulin is greatly reduced as a result.

Increasing Protein and Fiber

Increasing your consumption of fiber and protein are two more scientifically validated dietary recommendations for improved blood sugar management, in addition to concentrating your carb intake on low-GI meals.

One kind of indigestible carbohydrate that has major advantages for glucose regulation is fiber. It aids in reducing the rate at which digestible carbohydrates are absorbed, which lessens the postmeal spike in insulin and blood sugar. Foods high in fiber also help you feel fuller for longer.

Vegetables are a good source of fiber; the more, the better!

- Berries
- Avocados
- Seeds and nuts
- Pulses, beans, and lentils
- Whole grains
- Moderate servings of fruits low in sugar, such as citrus and apples

Achieving a minimum of 30-40 grams of fiber daily from these whole food sources may significantly enhance one's sensitivity to insulin.

Since protein provides consistent energy and has no effect on blood sugar levels, it is also crucial for correcting prediabetes. During weight reduction, dietary protein boosts metabolism while maintaining lean muscle mass.

Among the best sources of protein are eggs and poultry.

- Seafood and fish
- Yogurt and cottage cheese from Greece
- Seeds and nuts
- Lentils with beans

Incorporating lean protein into every meal, particularly breakfast, may help prevent blood sugar increases caused by carbohydrates and keep you full in between meals.

Generally, eating a diet centered on high-fiber, high-protein meals will fill you full with comparatively little calories and carbohydrates. This naturally promotes a calorie deficit for weight reduction when necessary, while also lowering the strain on your body to create insulin.

Good Fats and Portion Management

Healthy fats derived from whole food sources have no discernible effect on insulin or blood sugar levels, in contrast to processed carbohydrates and sugar. Insulin sensitivity may be further improved by substituting healthier fat sources for carb and protein sources that are higher in harmful saturated fats.

Healthy fat sources include avocados, olive oil, and avocado oil.

- - Almonds and their butters
- - Hemp, flax, and chia seeds
- - High-fat dairy items like cheese and plain Greek yogurt
- Fatty fish like mackerel, sardines, and salmon

Due to their high content of omega-3 polyunsaturated and monounsaturated fatty acids, these meals may help lower insulin resistance.

It's crucial to maintain total fat consumption between 20 and 35 percent of daily caloric intake, however. Overindulging in fats may decrease insulin sensitivity, yet overindulging in fats encourages weight gain. It's best to include good fats from entire foods without going overboard.

Speaking of excess, a crucial part of any diet for prediabetes is reducing your total portion sizes. Controlling calories and losing weight is a very effective way to reverse insulin resistance.

Even a little daily calorie reduction of 500–750 calories will help you lose weight steadily and sustainably while still enabling you to consume enough protein and other nutrients. This is made simpler with little tricks like eating slowly until satiated rather than full, foregoing seconds, and utilizing smaller dishes.

Moreover, low-calorie meal substitutions increase nutrients while using less calories:

- Eating fresh berries or apple slices with nut butter instead of crackers or cereal bars; substituting zucchini noodles or cauliflower rice for conventional rice or pasta;
- Giving baked or grilled lean proteins precedence over fried or fatty meat portions.

You may progressively lose weight while balancing your blood sugar levels by eating nutrient-dense, high-fiber, high-protein meals with healthy fats and measuring quantities carefully. This food strategy works wonders when combined with consistent exercise to reverse prediabetes.

This chapter's dietary methods provide a flexible framework that can be adjusted to fit your tastes and way of life, all while achieving the ultimate aim of using food to reverse prediabetes, lower blood sugar, and reduce insulin resistance. In the next chapter, we will now go into the workout component.

Chapter 4:

Exercise for Prediabetes

Dietary modifications are essential for correcting prediabetes, but they shouldn't be the main priority. Another important therapeutic lifestyle strategy for enhancing glucose regulation and insulin sensitivity is exercise. In controlling and correcting prediabetes, regular physical exercise may be very beneficial when paired with a balanced, nutrient-dense diet.

This chapter will discuss the many advantages exercise has for people with prediabetes, examine the differences in the effects of resistance and aerobic training, and provide organized advice for creating a regimen you can stay with for long-term benefits.

Advantages of Physical Activity

Research keeps showing how effective exercise is in raising insulin sensitivity and lowering blood sugar in those with type 2 diabetes and prediabetes. Here are a few of the main advantages:

A Greater Sensitivity to Insulin
Insulin sensitivity is raised during exercise because working muscles can absorb glucose from the circulation more efficiently. Up to 72 hours after exercise, muscles continue to work on self-repairing and refueling, which might cause this elevated sensitivity.

Reduced Levels of Blood Sugar

A1C testing show that aerobic and resistance training both lower fasting blood sugar levels and enhance overall blood sugar management. Frequent exercise improves blood glucose-regulating metabolic mechanisms.

Loss of Weight and Diminished Belly Fat
Exercise aids in the loss of extra weight and visceral fat that is stored around the abdominal organs when paired with a diet low in calories. Even a little weight loss of 5–10% of body weight may correct prediabetes and greatly improve insulin sensitivity.

Enhanced Metabolic Rate and Physical Fitness
Exercise improves metabolism, lean muscle mass, and cardiovascular health by increasing the body's ability to use glucose as fuel. Prevention of diabetes and general health benefit greatly from this.

Decreased Inflammation

Increased insulin resistance is associated with systemic inflammation, which is reduced by physical exercise. Exercise reduces chronic inflammation, which is often linked to diabetes and obesity.

Enhanced Mood and Vitality

Exercise helps reduce the weariness and fogginess that often accompany insulin resistance by improving glucose management. It can also enhance mood by producing endorphins.

In a nutshell, exercise is a kind of "free medication" that helps your body regulate blood sugar levels again without the need of medications or other treatments. The advantages of resistance and aerobic exercise are complimentary.

Resistance vs. Aerobic Training

Any activity that engages your cardiovascular system for a prolonged amount of time is considered aerobic exercise. This improves how well your body utilizes oxygen by raising your respiratory and heart rates.

Your aerobic energy system is used during exercises like brisk walking, jogging or running, swimming, cycling, rowing, or sports. A regular stroll of thirty minutes may significantly increase insulin sensitivity.

The Department of Health advises prediabetics to engage in moderate aerobic exercise, such as brisk walking, for at least 150 minutes per week. You may be able to reach the goal in less time overall by engaging in more demanding aerobic exercises, such as running or swimming intervals.

Strength training, often known as resistance training, is another crucial element that supports aerobic activity. This includes using weights, resistance bands, your own body weight, or any other exercise that puts your muscles up against an opposing force.

Resistance exercise raises your muscles' sensitivity to insulin and their capacity to absorb glucose from the circulation by overloading and straining them. Your body uses more glucose as fuel when at rest if it has larger muscle mass.

For all major muscle groups, resistance training is advised by the Physical Activity Guidelines for Americans to be performed at least twice a week. Bodyweight strength training, Pilates, yoga, and weightlifting are a few examples of this.

The following are the greatest advantages of combining resistance and aerobic exercise to reverse prediabetes:

Aerobic exercise increases cardiovascular fitness, burns glucose, and aids in fat reduction. Resistance training increases muscle mass, which raises metabolic rate and insulin sensitivity.

A thorough program that integrates components of both training modalities enhances your functional strength and fitness and improves your glucose regulation.

Establishing a Workout Schedule

Now that you know how important it is to include both resistance and aerobic training, it's time to design an exercise program that you can maintain in order to reverse your prediabetes. Here are some pointers:

Build up gradually at first

To prevent injury or burnout, it's advisable to start off gently if you've never exercised regularly. Start with bodyweight exercises or gentle walking for ten to fifteen minutes, then progressively increase the duration. Pushing yourself too hard, too quickly, may result in severe muscular discomfort that throws off your routine.

Plan It Out

Writing down your workout schedule on your calendar increases the likelihood that it will become ingrained. Prior to the rigors of the day, most people feel that morning exercises are the simplest to maintain. Finding an evening session that works best for you is important.

Stir Things Up

Including a range of various resistance and aerobic workouts keeps you from becoming bored and uses your muscles in new ways. Maybe switch between fast walks, swimming, and riding. To target all main muscular groups, use bodyweight exercises, bands, and dumbbells.

Take a nap and recuperate.

Even while consistency is crucial, it's also critical to take regular days off to allow your body to heal, particularly after strenuous exercise. Think about taking a whole day off every week.

Request Assistance

Seek advice from experts like personal trainers or physical therapists if you're new to exercising or have medical constraints. They can help you choose the right exercise regimens and make sure you're using the right technique to prevent injuries.

Monitor Your Development

You're inspired to observe continuous progress over time when you track metrics like body weight, waist circumference, resting heart rate, and fitness indicators like how many pushups you can do.

Remain persistent and patient.

It takes committed lifestyle changes over weeks and months to reverse prediabetes, so don't give up if you don't notice benefits right away. Have faith that your efforts will be rewarded by sticking to your strategy religiously.

This workout regimen has the added advantage of improving general health in addition to reversing insulin resistance and prediabetes. As your fitness increases, you'll have more energy, sleep better, lower your risk of illness, and maybe even be able to minimize how much medicine you use.

Probably above all, developing an exercise routine gives you the self-assurance and responsibility to maintain the food and lifestyle adjustments required to permanently kick prediabetes. If you combine this commitment to exercise with the other tactics in this book, you can reverse your prediabetes.

Chapter 5:

Weight Management

One of the most effective therapies for curing prediabetes and avoiding type 2 diabetes if you are overweight or obese is to lose weight. Insulin resistance is mostly caused by excess body fat, particularly in the abdomen. But even a little weight loss may have a significant positive impact on your body's capacity to control blood sugar levels.

This chapter will discuss the significance of maintaining a healthy weight for the management of prediabetes, provide suggestions for realistic goal-setting for weight reduction, and offer methods for implementing lifestyle modifications that promote long-term success.

The Value of Losing Weight

Growing overweight is directly correlated with increased insulin resistance, according to a number of research. An individual's risk of developing prediabetes, type 2 diabetes, and metabolic dysfunction increases with their excess weight.

Compounds including free fatty acids, hormones, and inflammatory chemicals are released by excess adipose tissue (fat cells), and these substances have the direct ability to interfere with insulin's regular signaling pathways and function. Over time, these actions increase cells' resistance to insulin.

Visceral fat, which builds up around the organs in the abdomen, is especially dangerous because it contributes to insulin resistance. This viscous abdominal fat secretes chemicals that aggravate metabolic health and initiates systemic inflammation, functioning akin to an active endocrine organ.

Fortunately, overcoming insulin resistance and prediabetes may be greatly aided by shedding even 5–10% of your present body weight:

- In those with prediabetes, a mere 5-7% reduction in weight has been shown to reduce the risk of type 2 diabetes by more than 50%.

- For around three out of four persons, losing 7-10% of body weight may help bring blood sugar levels back to a normal, non-prediabetic range.

- A modest weight reduction of ten to fifteen pounds significantly lowers blood insulin levels and increases insulin sensitivity.

- As weight is lost, inflammatory markers and belly fat decrease together, improving blood sugar regulation.

Losing weight has a variety of effects on correcting prediabetes. As you lose more weight:

- Fatty acids and inflammatory substances decrease, decreasing obstacles to insulin synthesis
- Insulin receptors become more sensitive and effective
- Pancreatic beta cells may "reset" and resume normal insulin production

- Smaller fat cells are less metabolically active and disruptive

Achieving a healthy body weight reduces the risk of heart disease, stroke, several malignancies, and other chronic diseases made worse by excess weight in addition to avoiding type 2 diabetes.

Even while decreasing a large amount of weight has more advantages, if you are overweight, shedding even 5–10% of your body weight may be a crucial first step towards restoring your metabolic health. Most people can achieve this modest level of weight reduction.

Having Reasonable Objectives

Setting attainable targets specific to your situation will help you reap the most advantages of weight reduction for curing prediabetes. While it's desirable to work toward a goal weight that enables you to achieve a BMI in the "normal" range of 18.5-24.9, losing weight may have an influence at any level.

If you are overweight or obese, starting with a 5-7% weight loss from your present body weight is a suitable objective. That means a 200-pound individual would lose 10 to 14 pounds. Once you reach that milestone, you may then reassess and make new plans.

It's crucial to avoid starting with too high expectations, such as aiming to lose 3–4 pounds a week. Although drastic calorie cutting may achieve that pace of loss for a little while, it is exceedingly difficult to maintain over the long term and often results in weight cycling as old habits resurface.

One to two pounds of weight reduction per week may be safely and sustainably achieved with small daily calorie deficits of 500–750 and moderate lifestyle changes. With effort, you may feasibly lose 10 pounds at this rate in two to three months.

Make sure you pay attention to changes in body composition as well as the scale number. Waist circumference decreases may be more accurately measured using a tape measure to assess visceral fat loss. Strength training helps maintain muscle that increases metabolism while losing weight.

The secret is to create realistic, reasonably paced objectives that are specific to you and, if you reach them, to set new ones again. Keeping an ultimate goal in mind helps you stay motivated and gives you the flexibility to make smart adjustments as required.

Techniques for Sustainable Achievement

Although losing weight initially might be difficult, the true struggle for long-term success is to permanently alter the lifestyle choices and behaviors that first made it possible for extra weight to accumulate. Here are some tried-and-true methods for maintaining your weight reduction and reversing prediabetes:

Create a Dietary Deficit of Calories

For healthy weight loss, it is essential to consistently create a calorie deficit via portion-controlled, balanced diet. Pay attention to nutrient-dense, high-fiber, high-protein meals that help to balance blood sugar levels and increase satiety.

Exercise Frequently

A combination of aerobic and strength training exercises for 150–300 minutes a day may help you lose weight by boosting your metabolism, maintaining lean muscle mass, and using more glucose as fuel.

Make Protein Your Top Priority: Place a strong emphasis on obtaining 25–30% of your calories from lean, high-quality protein sources, such as Greek yogurt, fish, chicken, and lentils. Protein has minimal effect on blood sugar levels, promotes sensations of fullness, and stops muscle atrophy.

Maintain Hydration

It has been shown that getting enough water increases your feeling of fullness in between meals and speeds up your metabolism a little. To prevent overindulging, have a glass before meals and snacks.

Make Enough Sleep

Insulin resistance, overeating, obesity, and elevated hunger hormones have all been related to inadequate sleep length and quality. Make getting 7-9 hours of sleep every night a priority by developing healthy sleeping habits.

Control Your Stress

Practicing stress-reduction techniques such as yoga, meditation, and low-impact exercise might help avoid long-term increases in cortisol levels, which can lead to cravings and weight gain in the abdomen.

Weigh Frequently

Regular self-monitoring via daily or weekly weight monitoring, according to studies, improves awareness and adherence to the portion management and exercise routines necessary for long-term weight reduction.

Develop Assistance

Working with a certified health coach, joining a support group, or having an accountability partner may help you stay motivated and give direction as you overcome obstacles.

Honor significant anniversaries

Celebrate each 5–10 pounds gone or healthy habit you've mastered. This encouraging feedback gives one the drive to keep moving forward.

In the end, curing prediabetes and regaining your health requires a whole change in lifestyle, not simply a new diet. You'll be able to lose extra weight and keep it off permanently by practicing discipline with regard to healthy diet, consistent exercise, enough sleep, and other aspects of a balanced lifestyle.

Although losing weight might feel overwhelming at first, there is a clear path to success if you follow an organized strategy that permits a moderate pace and continuous improvement. As you begin to reap the significant advantages of improved glucose regulation and enhanced insulin sensitivity, you will be inspired to make these adjustments a permanent part of your lifestyle.

Chapter 6:

Stress Management

Managing your stress is crucial for curing prediabetes and regaining control over your blood sugar levels. Many of the beneficial measures you're doing with your diet and fitness regimen might be directly undermined by ongoing stress and inadequate coping strategies.

We will go into the science of how stress hormones affect glucose metabolism and insulin sensitivity in this chapter. You'll pick up a range of tried-and-true methods for body and mind relaxation. Additionally, you'll get helpful advice for enhancing the quality of your sleep, which is another essential step in lowering insulin resistance and stress.

Stress's Effects on Blood Sugar

While managing sporadic stresses is inevitable in life, putting off chronic stress might have detrimental effects on your metabolic health. Making stress management a habit is motivated by realizing these detrimental effects.

Your body releases hormones such as cortisol, epinephrine (adrenaline), glucagon, and growth hormone in response to an intensely stressful situation. Your sympathetic nervous system triggers a "fight-or-flight" response, giving you a surge of energy to either battle the perceived danger or run away.

Raising blood sugar levels is a step in this process that makes sure your muscles and cells have access to adequate glucose for fuel. It makes sense as a survival strategy for our ancestors who faced biological hazards like ravenous predators.

The challenge facing our contemporary society is that persistent psychological stresses such as demanding job schedules, financial hardships, challenging interpersonal dynamics, or unfavorable thinking patterns maintain this "on" state of flight-or-fight response. Your body eventually marinates in excessive doses of stress chemicals on a regular basis.

This protracted condition of imbalance over time might severely impair your body's capacity to control blood sugar:

High insulin levels are required to overcome this hormonal resistance, and the pancreas is unable to keep up, resulting in high blood glucose levels. Growth hormone opposes insulin and stimulates glucose production. Cortisol causes the liver to produce more glucose while making cells insulin resistant. Glucagon signals the liver to release stored glucose into the bloodstream.

Essentially, long-term stress sets up the ideal internal conditions for the onset of prediabetes, which then deteriorates as insulin resistance steadily increases.

However, stress's detrimental consequences don't end there. Raising cortisol levels causes desires for fatty, sugary meals and increases appetite—exactly the opposite of what you want when attempting to correct prediabetes with diet. Poor sleep is another typical result of stress, which exacerbates metabolic abnormalities.

It is obvious that even the finest diet and exercise plans to decrease blood sugar will be undermined if stress is still rife in your life. It is essential, not optional, to practice daily relaxation and build resilience against long-term stresses.

Techniques for Relaxation

Regularly practicing relaxation techniques enables you to physically offset your body's fight-or-flight stress reaction. Your parasympathetic "rest-and-digest" system may be deliberately engaged to regulate blood sugar and bring your body back into balance.

The following are some tried-and-true methods for triggering the relaxation response:

Inhaling deeply

Breathing gently and deeply for many minutes might have significant effects. Breathe in through your nose for four counts, allowing your stomach to expand completely. After pausing, gently release the breath via pressed lips six times. Your brain is signaled to relax by this.

Gradual Relaxation of the Muscles

One by one, the primary muscular groups are progressively tensed and subsequently relaxed using this approach. Your thoughts will unwind in tandem with your body. You may be guided through it using a free audio application.

Mindfulness and Meditation

Stress-relieving techniques, such as utilizing an app for meditation, watching YouTube videos, or just finding a quiet place, lower the hormone cortisol. Give it even five to ten minutes a day.

Yoga and Mild Stretching

Focused breathing and yoga asanas (postures) have a profoundly relaxing impact because of their mind-body link. Yoga that is restorative, yin, and gentle is a great way to decompress.

Relaxing Interests

Your mind may be stilled from rushing thoughts by engaging in "get in the zone" activities like knitting, drawing, gardening, carpentry, or even simple dishwashing.

Choosing relaxation techniques you will really love and maintain over time is essential.

Putting a time block on your calendar makes it more likely to occur every day.

Obtaining Restful Sleep

Reducing stress and increasing the quality of your sleep each night go hand in hand. Getting enough good-quality sleep is essential for maintaining insulin sensitivity and stable blood sugar levels.

Studies have shown a robust correlation between insufficient sleep and heightened insulin resistance. A little sleep deficit may affect blood sugar regulation and interfere with hormones that regulate hunger, which increases the desire for unhealthy meals.

Every night, try to obtain between seven and nine hours of good sleep. Even on the weekends, maintaining a regular sleep and wake schedule will help you get more restful sleep.

The following advice may help you sleep better:

- Create an ideal bedroom atmosphere that is cold, quiet, dark, and screen-free.
- Engage in a soothing ritual before bed, such as mild yoga, having a bath, reading, or easy stretches.
- Download an app or use white noise to block outside noises;
- Use blackout curtains or an eye mask to prevent ambient light;
- Limit alcohol and caffeine after 2-3 pm since they might disturb sleep cycles.

Even on weekends, go to bed and get up at around the same hours every day. Steer clear of heavy meals too soon before bed. After 20 minutes, if you still can't sleep, get up and engage in a soothing activity. Daily physical activity is recommended, but avoid doing strenuous exercise just before bed.

Sometimes it's easier said than done to get decent sleep, particularly if you have a sleep problem like sleep apnea or persistent insomnia. If you need assistance getting back on track with your sleep, don't be afraid to see a doctor.

Improved Blood Sugar equals Better Sleep
Good sleep is essential for controlling blood sugar levels as well as aiding in your body's recovery. Your body is better able to control

the release of hormones like growth hormone and insulin while you sleep.

Additionally, those who sleep well often have greater amounts of the hormone leptin, which regulates hunger and helps people feel full, and lower levels of inflammatory chemicals, which may lead to insulin resistance.

Conversely, chronic sleep loss raises insulin resistance, decreases hormones associated with fullness and appetite, increases inflammation, and increases the desire for sugary foods and beverages for rapid energy bursts.

Stress, hectic schedules, and unhealthy behaviors all contribute to decreased sleep length and quality, which is a recipe for worsening obesity and prediabetes. However, by making relaxation techniques a priority and creating healthy sleep habits, you may maximize your body's capacity to use insulin correctly and keep your blood sugar levels steady all day.

Reversing prediabetes and regaining your general health and vigor may be accomplished with a comprehensive strategy that combines stress management, getting enough sleep, and following the diet and exercise recommendations outlined in this book.

Chapter 7:

Supplements and Medications

For prediabetes to be naturally reversed, lifestyle modifications, exercise, and proper diet should be the main priorities. However, certain vitamins and drugs may also help. Based on the existing scientific information, this chapter will assist you in determining which dietary supplements could be useful. Additionally, you'll discover the range of drug choices available for the treatment of type 2 diabetes and prediabetes.

Above all, you'll get advice on how to collaborate closely with the physicians, nurses, dietitians, and other members of your healthcare team. The administration of vitamins and drugs safely and effectively needs expert supervision tailored to your unique circumstances. Now let's get started!

Assessing Nutraceutical Supplements

The supplement business is rife with greatly overstated claims and no oversight of the effectiveness or safety of its products. When taken as directed, some vitamins, minerals, herbs, and other substances do, in fact, seem to have some real promise for enhancing insulin sensitivity and helping to treat prediabetes.

The following are some of the most intriguing supplements to talk to your physician about:

Chrome

This mineral is involved in the metabolism of fats and carbohydrates. By increasing cellular glucose absorption, chromium picolinate and high-molecular weight chromium yeast may improve insulin sensitivity. Research suggests that it may reduce A1C and blood sugar levels, particularly when used in conjunction with medicine.

Lipoic Acid Alpha

Antioxidant ALA, which the body naturally produces, has been shown to decrease blood sugar levels and lessen insulin resistance. It could also aid in the management of diabetic neuropathy problems. Consult your physician regarding appropriate dosage.

magnesium

A magnesium deficit is seen in up to 50% of individuals with type 2 diabetes, which exacerbates insulin resistance and metabolic syndrome. Additions of taurate, chloride, or magnesium glycinate may enhance lipid profiles and insulin sensitivity.

Cinnamon: In prediabetics and diabetics, extracts from this spice have shown promise in lowering fasting blood glucose levels, raising A1C, and boosting antioxidant status. Seek for supplements that have their polyphenol content standardized.

Berberine

This substance found in plants like Oregon grape may have effects similar to those of metformin treatment, including lowering blood sugar, decreasing inflammation, and enhancing insulin sensitivity. For most people, berberine presents a lesser risk than medicines.

It's important to do due diligence on high-quality supplements from reliable companies that have undergone independent testing for purity and efficacy. There are plenty of contaminated or filler-filled supplements on the market.

You may get advice on appropriate amounts for your unique requirements from your doctor or dietician. They can also tell you if some supplements should be taken continuously or in cycles. Never take more supplements than is advised or mix supplements without a doctor's approval.

Maintaining realistic expectations about supplements is also crucial. Compared to pharmaceuticals, the majority of their effects on prediabetes are mild, despite their promising nature. They should not completely replace other lifestyle modifications; rather, they should support them.

Options for Medication

Nutrition, exercise, and weight control alone are often insufficient for many individuals with prediabetes to lower blood sugar levels to a normal, healthy range. It could be necessary to use prescription drugs, at least temporarily.

Medication for prediabetes is most often administered as metformin, which belongs to the biguanide medicine class. Metformin mainly acts by making cells more sensitive to insulin and lowering the quantity of glucose the liver produces.

Research indicates that when paired with diet and exercise, metformin may dramatically reduce the chance of developing type 2 diabetes by 31% over a 3-year period when compared to a placebo. Additionally, it could protect blood arteries and the heart.

Over time, potential side effects such as nausea, bloating, diarrhea, and a metallic taste usually go away. Metformin is typically inexpensive, safe, and well-tolerated when taken as directed by a doctor. In addition, other drugs could be administered in tandem with:

Sulfonylureas: These induce the production of more insulin by the pancreas. Glyburide, glimepiride, and glipizide are a few examples. may result with periods of low blood sugar and weight gain.

Meglitinides: These fast-acting medications, which include nateglinide and repaglinide, also cause the pancreas to produce short-term drops in blood sugar levels after meals. entail a risk of weight gain and hypoglycemia as well.

Alpha-glucosidase inhibitors: Drugs such as miglitol and acarbose prevent the absorption of starches and carbs, hence reducing the rise in blood sugar that occurs after meals. Diarrhea, bloating, and gas are typical adverse effects.

Thiazolidinediones (TZDs): Pioglitazone and rosiglitazone are examples of medications in this family that increase insulin sensitivity in cells. They have adverse consequences such as weight gain and an elevated risk of fractures or congestive heart failure.

GLP-1 Opponents - Medication administered intravenously, such as semaglutide and liraglutide, imitates the actions of gut hormones that promote insulin release while inhibiting the generation of glucagon and delaying the emptying of the stomach. may aid with weight reduction as well. Show promise for prediabetes, but are more often used for type 2 diabetes.

Metformin, together with diet, exercise, and/or medication, may often be used as a potent multi-pronged strategy to reverse prediabetes and lower the risk of developing diabetes. The best routine will include close observation of your blood sugar levels and honest dialogue with your physician.

collaborating with your medical group

For effective management of your prediabetes, it is essential to work closely with a trained healthcare team, regardless of whether you use prescription medications, vitamins, injectable medicines, or none of the above. Physicians, endocrinologists, registered dietitians, pharmacists, diabetes educators, and any other healthcare providers who work with you fall under this category.

Your whole medical history, test findings, current prescriptions and supplements, and any lifestyle choices that could be affecting your health should all be shared with your specialists. It's also critical to be open about following their advice.

Never be reluctant to inquire! It's critical that you comprehend everything about your treatment plan, including the rationale behind any recommended drugs or supplements, any side effects to be aware of, and how to take them correctly. Your group is there to help and educate you.

Above all, remember that you are in charge of your own health path. Prescribers provide advice, but you have the last say after considering all the options. You are free to choose the course that seems most relevant to you.

But intentionally stopping or changing medicine without their permission may be quite dangerous, particularly when it comes to diabetic meds that affect insulin levels. Ask about other possibilities and be upfront about any issues you may have about medicine suggestions.

Third-party lab testing may detect potentially hazardous components in supplements, such as heavy metals, PCBs, poisons, etc. Your team may be able to provide trustworthy product suggestions.

Ultimately, your care team for prediabetes is here to support you and is prepared to provide advice as needed. You may assist your lifestyle in reversing insulin resistance and restoring your metabolic health by collaborating to choose the best supplement and pharmaceutical regimen.

Chapter 8:

Building Habits

It takes much more than simply understanding the proper food and lifestyle choices to reverse prediabetes. The key to long-lasting transformation is to radically alter deeply established patterns of eating, exercising, managing stress, and other behaviors. In the absence of forming enduring habits, transient drive eventually wanes.

This chapter delves into tried-and-true behavior modification concepts to help you rewire your behaviors for improved metabolic health. You'll discover typical roadblocks that often impede advancement and how to prepare for them. Additionally, you'll learn tactics for meal planning and preparation to ensure that your diet is successful.

Achieving a long-lasting adjustment in lifestyle takes time and effort. However, if you regularly put these ideas into practice, you'll have the mental structure and useful resources needed to make your health objectives become second nature.

Principles of Behavior Change

Decades of behavioral science study have been conducted on the psychological factors that influence human habits, both the creation of new ones and the breaking of existing ones. The following are a few of the most effective guidelines to follow:

Make It Clearly Visible

It is more probable that intended new behaviors will materialize when they are more widely known and understood. This may involve arranging your exercise gear and shoes the night before, putting fresh food in the refrigerator at eye level, or planning workouts with reminders on your calendar.

Make it Eye-Catching

Habits that are linked to happiness or advantages we appreciate will drive us more. Try to find methods to make routines more enticing, such as imagining the accomplishment you will feel from adhering to the plan, discovering new, nutritious foods that pique your interest, or listening to upbeat music while working out.

Make it simple.

New behaviors are much more likely to be continuously repeated when they are easy to start. Reduce obstacles by organizing your meals ahead of time, joining a nearby gym, or clearing your house of alluring junk food to help you make healthier choices automatically.

Make it fulfilling

Our innate need is for routines that provide us measurable outcomes, encourage us, and give us a sense of accomplishment. Measuring your body's changes, fitness advancements, or weight reduction all serve as gratifying sources of encouragement to go forward. Celebrating little victories along the road also helps.

Use these guidelines to gradually develop behaviors like as getting enough sleep, controlling your stress, exercising more throughout the day, and resisting sugar cravings. Reframe your thoughts, make adjustments to your surroundings, and get encouraging feedback to help you stick to your new routines.

Modest Changes Compound

It might be intimidating to consider completely changing your way of life, which will surely result in emotions of deprivation, frustration, and perhaps giving up. For this reason, experts advise beginning with modest, manageable behavioral changes and allowing them to gain traction gradually.

In only a single year, a 37% improvement is achieved with a daily minor change of 1%. And a 37% improvement in your stress levels, sleep patterns, food, and physical activity would undoubtedly aid in the reversal of prediabetes.

A few instances of 1% shifts are:

- Including a portion of vegetables in one meal a day;
- Replacing one sugary drink with water
- Walking around the block for ten minutes; (5) using an app for guided meditation; and (6) preparing some of your meals in advance for the next day.

Starting anywhere you can realistically is the aim. Small enough to be easily maintained, even on your busiest or least motivated days, are the new habits to aim for. After a few weeks or months, reevaluate to look for chances to change by an extra 1%.

By using a stepwise approach, you avoid feeling overpowered and may gradually see the transformative impact of small, incremental behavior adjustments.

Overcoming Difficulties

It is expected that new lifestyle habits may encounter challenges. However, being aware of the most typical traps and having a strategy to avoid them is rather effective.

Lack of motivation and procrastination

It is certain that there may be days when you will not want to put in the effort necessary to keep up your new habits. This is acceptable and typical. However, delaying makes it far more difficult to get started again. Include an exercise partner, schedule routines at regular intervals, or make public posts about your objectives on social media to increase accountability.

Emotional Consumption

Even the best-intentioned attempts to cope with negative feelings such as stress, worry, boredom, despair, etc. by turning to food may quickly backfire. Establish coping mechanisms like as writing, contacting a friend, practicing meditation, or taking a stroll when you sense the need to eat.

Social Customs

If unhealthy practices are the norm in your social circle, family, and daily life, it may be difficult to stick with new behaviors. Never be scared to suggest politely that someone support your aims or to establish reasonable limits. They could be inspired by you too. Take charge of the things that you can manage.

Journey and Typical Disruptions

While some disruptions to your habits are unavoidable, they often have the potential to utterly derail you. Plan ahead for how you'll maintain habit adherence during travel or schedule changes by organizing your meals, creating an exercise regimen, acquiring any necessary equipment, etc.

All-or-Nothing Thinking: Avoid self-defeating thoughts that lead to self-sabotage since perfection is unachievable. Don't let occasional deviations from your planned habits lead to a complete return to your previous behaviors. Accept it, give yourself a pass, and go on to your very next decision.

Your routines will not become huge derailments from tiny setbacks if you have a strategy in place to handle these barriers.

Preparing and Organizing Meals

Probably the most important step in naturally correcting prediabetes is to eat a balanced, blood sugar-stabilizing diet. However, maintaining a balanced diet without a meal plan and without at least some previous preparation is quite difficult.

Organizing Meals

Having a weekly meal plan, or at least one for the next few days, eliminates any uncertainty and decision fatigue when it comes to eating. It makes sure you receive the right amount of lean proteins, healthy fats, fruits, vegetables, and other kinds of carbohydrates high in fiber.

Additionally, it simplifies portioning out meals and facilitates selecting the correct items. Create meal plans specifically for controlling prediabetes with the help of apps and internet resources. But don't make things too difficult!

Preparing Meals

Once your meal plan is established, ahead-of-time component preparation really makes all the difference. It offers alternatives that are ready to eat when hunger hits, while also drastically cutting down on the time and work required to prepare meals.

A few fundamentals of meal prep:

• Clean, chop, and divide raw vegetables into snack bags.

Make individual servings of snacks and sides like hard-boiled eggs, homemade trail mix, hummus, etc.; Cook large batches of proteins like chicken breasts, fish, ground turkey, etc.; Parboil starches like potatoes, rice, or pasta to finish cooking later; Portion out and freeze part of an extra-large recipe for heat-and-eat leftovers.

You may set yourself up for success all week long by dedicating even an hour or two on weekends or days off to effective meal planning. Make sure you have an abundance of grab-and-go alternatives in your pantry and fridge to make unhealthy grabs far less enticing.

Naturally, life continues to occur. There will be days when food planning and rigorous adherence to your schedule don't go as planned. That's OK; strive for an 80/20 ratio, in which you carry out your plan for the most part but leave room for social gatherings and the odd outing to accommodate yourself.

Establishing a conducive atmosphere for achievement is crucial. It's much simpler to build healthy eating habits and overcome temptations when you have well-portioned, readily-prepared meals that fit into your day.

Forming habits is not about punishing yourself or leading an endlessly deprived life. It's about creating routines and little, significant changes that, over time, put your behaviors and health on autopilot. Reversing your prediabetes becomes a fulfilling journey of long-lasting lifestyle modification when you have the correct mindset and strategy in place.

Chapter 9:

Tracking Progress

You've completely changed the way you eat, included exercise into your daily routine, and devoted yourself to stress management. Everything is set up to permanently reverse your prediabetes. But how do you know whether all of your effort is being appreciated?

Every health and lifestyle change requires careful recording and monitoring of your progress. It offers the impartial, data-driven feedback loop you need to make sure you're still moving in the correct direction toward your objectives. It is also essential since it lets you commemorate accomplishments and concrete victories along the route.

The most important biometrics to regularly monitor as a person with prediabetes are covered in this chapter. You'll get instructions on the best testing procedures and intervals. Additionally, you'll discover how to reinterpret "slip-ups" using progress monitoring as a motivational framework.

Checking Your Blood Sugar

The main statistic you should definitely keep an eye on is your blood sugar levels, as that's the whole point of correcting prediabetes. The best approach to assess if your diet, exercise, sleep patterns, stress reduction, and other lifestyle changes are having the intended effect is to take regular at-home glucose tests.

As a baseline, your doctor could ask you to undergo a fasting blood sugar test first thing in the morning before eating. Alternatively, they can advise you to take a test one to two hours after eating in order to gauge how effectively your body is absorbing glucose.

Purchasing a high-quality glucose meter and a enough supply of test strips is a prudent decision, since they provide continuous, real-time input on how certain meals, activities, and other factors impact your individual blood sugar response. Apps or manual logbooks make tracking easier.

Testing your blood sugar on a regular basis can help you recognize ideal patterns and help you immediately determine whether certain decisions lead to unwanted variations or long-term spikes. You can make course corrections more quickly as a result.

In addition to daily self-monitoring, it's essential to do lab testing on occasion:

A1C Measurements

The A1C test calculates the proportion of glycated (sugar-coated) hemoglobin in your red blood cells to determine your typical blood sugar levels over the previous two to three months. An A1C of 5.7% to 5.9% is regarded as normal, while 5.7% to 6.4% is indicative of prediabetes.

The objective is to reduce your A1C to less than 5.7% by making dietary and lifestyle adjustments. Every three to six months, your doctor will want this test to be performed.

Glucose Plasma Fasting

After an 8-hour fast, a quick blood test determines if your overnight fasting glucose levels are within a safe range of less than 100 mg/dL. Findings between 100 and 125 mg/dL suggest prediabetes.

Test for Oral Glucose Tolerance

This test measures your blood sugar two hours after you consume a sweet beverage and again after an overnight fast. Less than 140 mg/dL at 2 hours is considered normal, however 140–199 mg/dL is indicative of prediabetes.

Together with regular self-monitoring with a glucose meter, these routine lab tests provide a thorough understanding of how well your body uses insulin and maintains stable blood sugar levels. You can control your prediabetes as well as your doctor can with the use of this data.

Keeping an Eye on Additional Metrics

On your path to reversing prediabetes, controlling your blood sugar levels should come first, but other health indicators also need careful observation. After all, a number of conditions, like being overweight, being physically unfit, having high blood pressure, and others, aggravate insulin resistance.

A few crucial parameters to consistently monitor in addition to your blood glucose levels are:

Body Mass and Fat

Achieving a weight loss goal of 5–10% of your total body weight will significantly improve insulin sensitivity and return blood sugar control to normal. Track your weight reduction efforts weekly or monthly using a scale. Positive changes are also shown by measurements of body fat percentage and waist circumference.

Blood Pressure

It's advisable to regularly check your blood pressure at home or with a doctor since both high blood pressure (hypertension) and low blood pressure (hypotension) might make blood sugar management more difficult. Blood pressure is also measured by several glucose meters.

Markers of Fitness

Observing gains in your strength, aerobic capacity, endurance, and other performance indicators encourages you to continue working out regularly. It also indicates that you are making progress toward improving metabolic health. Make use of exercise monitoring apps or fitness assessments.

Life Quality

The "unseen" effects of your prediabetes reversal journey may become clearer if you monitor quality of life indicators like as your energy, mood, stress perception, and sleep patterns. These effects are difficult to fully measure. Keeping a daily notebook might be helpful in seeing trends.

Lipids in Blood

Every six to twelve months, you should have your doctor examine your cholesterol levels, including LDL, HDL, and triglycerides. This will verify that your diet and exercise regimen are improving this important indicator of cardiovascular health.

nutrient concentrations

Getting routine nutritional testing for indicators like vitamin D, iron, B12, and magnesium guarantees you aren't becoming deficient in important vitamins and minerals, especially if your eating habits have changed significantly.

In the end, prediabetes-related elevated blood sugar and insulin resistance affect every part of the body, not just one particular measurement. Keeping an eye on a wide range of pertinent biometrics provides you and your medical team with the whole picture required for efficient treatment.

Honoring Achievements

Being blind to the accomplishments that have already been made in favor of the difficult journey ahead is a definite way to burn out and feel cheated. To maintain motivation, it is essential to acknowledge and appreciate every milestone and "small win," regardless of their size.

Establishing clear objectives and implementing a rewards system encourages good behavior and trains your brain to seek the satisfaction that comes from reaching goals. It makes use of the behavior change tenets of habit satisfaction and consistent reinforcement.

It's not necessary to applaud dramatic progress. Perhaps over the last two days, your morning fasting glucose has dropped to an all-time low. Or you succeeded in meditating every day for a whole week. Recognizing anything that moves you closer to your objectives is worthwhile.

Include incentives in your daily routine:

- Purchase the new training shirt you've been eyeing if you work out five days this week.
- Treat yourself to a massage or other indulgence once you shed your first five pounds.
- A new kitchen tool is awarded for completing four weeks of meal preparation.
- Taking a weekend getaway is equivalent to obtaining 8 hours of sleep every night for a whole month.

Excessive prizes are not necessary; the real power is in the act of celebration, not in the material "prize." It strengthens the identities, routines, and behaviors you are trying to establish as long-term modifications to your way of life.

This attitude of appreciating non-scale triumphs may be applied to more than simply individual accomplishments:

- Honestly recorded exceeding your daily calorie allotment? Honor your self-awareness!
- Completely destroyed your exercise because of a crazy schedule? Celebrate continuing to work hard and show up!
- Made a mistake and drank too much alcohol with pals? Rejoice when you get back on track the next day!

Refocusing on the broad picture while acknowledging that mistakes and faults are part of the process leads to a more sustainable and healthy way of thinking. It's a welcome change from poisonous "all-or-nothing" mentality, which interprets every mistake as total failure.

Real lifestyle change is a long-term process that calls for a great deal of perseverance, fortitude, and self-compassion. Those quick massages, kitchen toys, or evenings out serve as your go-to "bright spots" that will keep you moving forward.

However, by consistently acknowledging your biometric monitoring progress—such as decreased fasting blood sugar, reduced waist circumference, increased energy, etc.—you personally feel the significant results of all your hard work. It's your constant reminder that, little by little, you're taking back control of prediabetes.

CONCLUSION

Congratulations! You've made it to the finish! When you close this massive book, you will have started a whole new chapter in your life. You now have access to all the information, techniques, and inspiration need to reverse your prediabetes.

You now have a thorough grasp of the physiological aspects of prediabetes, including how insulin resistance and dysregulated blood sugar levels may cause a host of secondary health problems, including as cancer, neuropathy, and type 2 diabetes. You understand that prediabetes is a critical turning point that calls for action rather than indolence.

However, this work is about much more than just understanding the issue. You now have a clear understanding of the solution's plan as well, which is a multimodal strategy focused on stress management, physical activity enhancement, smart dietary treatments, and sleep quality optimization. These pillars were dissected in great depth, providing particulars about:

Putting a focus on nutrient-dense, high-fiber whole foods; reducing consumption of processed sugar and carbohydrates; and adding extra lean protein and healthy fats

• Choosing a workout regimen that fits your schedule; using stress-reduction methods like yoga and meditation; creating a regular nighttime schedule for restful sleep; enlisting the assistance and direction of your healthcare team; and setting attainable objectives to progressively create enduring habits

This comprehensive combination of long-term, sustainable lifestyle changes targets the underlying causes of prediabetes by reducing body weight, raising insulin sensitivity, resetting hormonal balances, and eventually reestablishing blood sugar homeostasis. You may regain control over your metabolic health using empirically validated methods rather than short cuts, fad diets, or miracle drugs.

You have been given a detailed plan for implementing each element strategically in these chapters, which include:

Making the switch to a diet higher in protein and fat and lower in carbohydrates;

developing a well-rounded aerobic and strength exercise regimen; including daily relaxation and stress-reduction techniques; and using sleep hygiene techniques to ensure enough rest and recuperation

Using the concepts of habit development to create long-lasting change; monitoring relevant biometrics such as weight, glucose, and fitness levels; acknowledging accomplishments and appropriately interpreting "slip-ups";

When used together, these components create a base that progressively changes your whole way of living to one that is sustainable and health-promoting. Unlike fleeting motivational spikes that eventually fade, these consistent behaviors permanently change your thought patterns.

Prediabetes is no longer permitted to deteriorate and push you closer to type 2 diabetes, chronic disease, and a reduced quality of life by continuously increasing insulin resistance. You no longer accept as your new normal persistent lethargy, fogginess in your head, unwavering weight increase, and unsettling blood test results.

From this turning point on, you are taking charge and actively reversing those harmful trends with nutrition, physical activity, stress reduction, and all the other self-care techniques necessary for vigorous life. You're taking back command. You're starting again in the direction of a healthier metabolism.

Will you have to be persistent for it to work? Indeed. A true change in lifestyle is never "easy" in the conventional sense. There will be days when your drive wanes, your discipline falters, and the allure of reverting to old behaviors beckons. Fighting against engrained behaviors will inevitably lead to the occasional difficulty.

But that same friction serves as a reminder that you're working hard and on worthwhile projects. You're gradually eliminating the habits that contributed to your prediabetes. By methodically constructing new brain pathways and entrenched behaviors, you're ultimately going to make healthy living seem as natural as brushing your teeth.

Beyond just correcting prediabetes, maintaining a healthy lifestyle centered on enough physical exercise, balanced diet, reduced stress, and good sleep has many benefits:

Increased physical stamina, strength, and mobility; improved mood and self-confidence from achieving objectives; improved attention and mental clarity as brain fog lifts; and a higher quality of life free from chronic illnesses like neuropathy, fatty liver disease, or even cancer

Consistency with the techniques in this book will have a cascading impact on all aspects of your well-being: financial, relational, professional, and emotional. Never undervalue the multiplicative effects that come from taking back your physical vigor.

Accept that this is a journey as a result. When it comes to health and fitness, there is no "finish line". However, you now have the awareness, the vision, and the practical strategy needed to divert off one problematic course and onto a much better one for your long-term well-being.

Through these pages, you have made the vital first step in fully educating yourself. The last step is to apply this lesson consistently every day to create lifelong habits. Tracking meals, recording exercises, and practicing meditation all add up to significant changes in metabolism.

Thus, see this as a starting point rather than a conclusion. A clear road map for curing prediabetes and reducing your risk of type 2 diabetes has created momentum. Moving forward, the focus will be on consistently executing daily tasks while being resilient in the face of life's inevitable disappointments.

Have faith in the procedure. Have faith in the underlying good reasoning of using tried-and-true methods for stress reduction, exercise, diet, and sleep optimization on a regular basis. Stable blood sugar levels, weight loss, and increased energy are the outcomes you want, and they come from consistent work.

Above all, however, have faith in yourself. You are now in possession of the information. You are the one who defines what it is to live completely and vigorously. And you've made the decision to stop taking declining health lying down.

Over time, you will be propelled gradually in the correct path by your own determination, dedication, and tenacity. You now have everything you need to complete this quest successfully.

Let me conclude by saying this: this is not only about reversing prediabetes. And that's just the start. Regaining the finest version of yourself for many years to come is really what you're looking for. A rendition full of vitality, self-assurance, and an actualized love of life.

Every piece of effort you put in starting now will pay off in the future when you become a rejuvenated version of yourself.

So take a brave move towards adopting these new lifestyle practices. Never take your foot off the gas as you tirelessly pursue optimum health. This is something you can handle!